INTERMITTENT FASTING

A Nutritionist's Guide to Lose Belly Fat Whilst Eating What You Want - It's Simpler Than You Think

SIMON KELLER

TABLE OF CONTENTS

INTRODUCTION

Can you really have your cake and eat it?

Excuse the pun, but with intermittent fasting you really can. I know this sounds like an exceptional claim, but in my opinion, this way of eating really is the panacea to virtually all human ailments...

Want to lose weight? Want to put on muscle? Want to cleanse your body? Want to sleep better? Want to have more energy? These are just a handful of benefits which I, and virtually everyone I put onto an intermittent fasting program has achieved.

How can this be? The trick is eating the way we evolved to eat. When we would go for long periods throughout the day (often the entire day) before we gathered or killed our next meal. Eating every 2-3 hours was rarely an option back on the African Savannah's, so we adapted to dealing with our nutrition in a much more efficient way.

We call it intermittent fasting today. Our ancestors would have just considered it a normal day. They certainly did just fine, and even thrived with this method of nutritional timing. Not out of choice, but out of circumstance.

What is not to like? You are essentially only eating two or three large meals a day. You spend less time cooking/preparing food, less time actually eating meals. You can eat big satiating meals you like, without constricting either what you are eating or the amount of calories of those meals.

I get asked all of the time what this intermittent fasting "diet"is all about. But in truth, this is the wrong way of looking at it. Diets are fads. Intermittent fasting is a way of more appropriately scheduling your eating patterns. It's a way of more intelligently scheduling your meals to get the most from them.

I have tried to summarize the science as much as I can to prevent this guide from becoming an overly technical white paper on the subject. My aim is to give you an overview of the benefits, whilst still referring to research. However I want to give you the practical tips and techniques to best implement this method of eating for best effect in your own life.

My Credentials

Before we get into the nitty-gritty of intermittent fasting, it's probably a good idea for me to explain exactly who I am, and why you should even bother listening to me in the first place. Yes I have the undergraduate in anatomy and physiology, and the master's degree in nutrition from Birmingham University in the UK.

However my main focus over the past 10 years has been on the practical implications of human performance. I now focus much more on the results of these principles in the real world, compared to my previous life of studying endless research papers on the academic side of the subject.

This includes everything from human movement to dietary considerations. What set of variables is most optimal for both myself, and the clients I now coach and mentor within my specialized training and wellness complex here in London.

Not everyone is the same, however there is a surprising amount of overlap when it comes to human physiology. With a few minor age, gender and genetic variations aside, we are all working with pretty much the same metabolic machinery. You just need to know how to get the most out of it.

So why am I such an expert on intermittent fasting? As I mentioned, I studied a wide range of topics within the field of cardio/respiratory physiology and nutrition whilst at university. This formed my base understanding of these subjects and how they fit together within a biological sense. However I have since put these academic theories and principles to the test in the real world. To really see what works and what doesn't with regards to completing the health and fitness puzzle.

I have undertook a journey of personal development and experimentation when it comes to human performance on myself first and foremost. I like to consider myself somewhat of a guinea pig when it comes to the physiological principles I test. I can then advise my clients on the best course of action for them.

The result of all this research has lead to me getting paid large sums to educate and train business professionals, athletes etc. However I still only have time to focus on a handful of clients at any one time. This is why I have switched to writing and publishing more work on these subjects, in order to educate as many people as I can, at a fraction of the cost of my one-on-one coaching.

Everything from devising peoples workout routines to managing their eating plans. From providing motivational and psychological guidance to lifestyle tips. I like to provide everything as a holistic approach to human performance. Because lets face it, we don't live out our lives in nice compartmentalized boxes. Everything blends into one, you have to up your efforts across the board to reap the full benefits of a healthy body and mind.

So now that you know a little more about me, let's dive in. The following chapters will teach you everything you need to know about intermittent fasting. What the theories are behind the science, and how you can best implement them into your own life for the amazing results IF can bring. This is one adjustment you can make which will have a big difference in your life. So get ready to give this a try, I promise you it will be worth it.

PART 1: INTERMITTENT FASTING - BASIC PRINCIPLES

CHAPTER 1: IT MAKES SENSE - THE SCIENCE BEHIND FASTING

"In a fast, the body tears down its defective parts and then builds anew when eating is resumed"

(Herbert M.Shelton)

The term intermittent fasting (IF) simply refers to the practice of not eating for extended periods of time throughout the day. As I mentioned within the introduction to this book, the concept is something that humans have been doing since our hunter gatherer ancestors inhabited the planet.

Today humans fast for a variety of reasons such as religious purposes, following certain rituals, food scarcity or simply sleeping. However regardless of culture and circumstance, the growing body of evidence and research is providing greater evidence to suggest that everybody should be partaking in some form of fasting throughout their day/week.

Hippocrates, the father of modern medicine, supported the practice of fasting and prescribed it to his patients. He suggested that, "To eat when you are sick, is to feed your illness." The same belief was held by other great thinkers throughout history, which include Plutarch, a Greek historian, Plato, and Aristotle. They all promoted fasting over the use of medicines.

"I fast for greater physical and mental efficiency"

(Plato)

It is part of human nature to stop eating when sick. This instinct is known as the physician within every human. If you have ever experienced over eating in the past, you will understand that it does more harm than good. A person tends to feel lethargic when full. Excess blood is directed to your digestive system and diverted away from vital organs including the brain. This is bad news if speed of body and mind is desirable.

So what are the reasons why so many people are reverting back to this type of lifestyle today? The two main considerations are body recomposition (I.e. fat loss/muscle gain) and the health benefits fasting can bring. I will get into these in greater depth within the following chapters, however here is an overview of both of these main benefits of IF:

#1 Weight Loss

IF helps you lose weight plain and simple. This process will naturally occur due to simply eating fewer meals. In addition to the reduction in overall daily calories, IF also boosts the hormones which aid in facilitating weight loss. As you go along with this style of eating, the levels of growth hormone production will also increase, as well as the concentration of norepinephrine in your system. You will also have lower insulin levels which will boost the breakdown of fats in your system. As your body gets used to the rhythms of IF, the body adapts and devises ways to use fats for energy more efficiently.

Even short-term fasting is effective in boosting a person's metabolic rate by up to 14 percent. This will allow you to burn more calories at a faster rate. A review of the scientific literature in 2014 found that IF is capable of helping a person lose up to 8 percent of his/her weight in just 3 to 24 weeks.

Another great benefit of IF is that the majority of the body fat a person will lose is around the belly area or the visceral fat. This fat is harmful as it builds up in and around the spaces of vital internal organs, such as the intestines and stomach. It produces toxins, including cytokines which reduces your sensitivity to insulin and increases your risk of heart disease. Cytokines can also worsen inflammation which increases your chances of certain cancers, especially those of the pancreas, colon, and esophagus.

Belly fat is a problem not only for overweight or obese people, but also for otherwise healthy individuals. This is due to the fat not only being stored as subcutaneous deposits I.e. beneath the skin, but also the internal organs as I mentioned above. However for most people aesthetics and physical appearance are the driving factor for wanting to lose weight (fat).

IF increases the propensity of your system to burn fat after it experiences a significant drop in the levels of insulin, and a boost in the levels of your growth hormone. The latter will also aid in building lean tissue which will further increase the fat burning potential of the person, as muscle is metabolizing energy substrates even whilst you sleep.

#2 Health Benefits

The first health component of IF is that it activates certain cellular repair processes, such as the removal of waste material. During the fasting period, your cells initiate autophagy or the "waste removal" process. As the cells break down, they metabolize the broken proteins in your body. When this process continues, your body will have more protection against various diseases, including most forms of cancer.

Cancer is a result of the uncontrolled growth of the cells. IF works by improving your metabolism, which results in a lower overall chance of developing such cancers in the first place. The studies done in this regard have largely been performed on animals, but the findings indicate promise for us too. Human cancer patients who follow the IF way of eating have shown a greater propensity to stave off cancer growth as well as reducing the effects of chemotherapy if they are undergoing treatment.

Another big consideration with regards to IF, is that it reduces oxidative stress, which is a major cause of chronic diseases. In fact oxidation is the only reason our bodies age in a physiological sense, and increased oxidative stress just speeds up this aging process. Although we can't escape this process, as oxygen is a critical component of the energy producing mechanisms within the cells, even when we are resting. However IF can reduce these levels as the person is consuming and metabolizing fewer energy substrates due to the overall reduction in caloric intake.

Essentially what is happening in the body during the oxidation process is the production of free radicals. These are atoms which are missing an electron is their out shell which can be highly destructive to the cells of the body. They will bump into healthy cells as they travel and steal these electrons to complete their structure, hence quickening the aging process and chronic disease formation.

You bodies natural defense system against this damage comes in the form of antioxidants such as vitamin C & E, which diffuse these destructive free radicals by donating an extra election in their out shell. This is especially important with regards to molecules in your system, such as DNA and brain tissue.

"Intermittent fasting enhances the ability of nerve cells to repair DNA"

(Mark Mattson - Neuroscientist)

IF is also highly effective in lowering insulin resistance and your blood sugar levels, which can greatly reduce your risk of Type 2 diabetes. There are studies which indicate that the fasting blood sugar of a person on this kind of diet, can be reduced by up to 6 percent, and fasting levels of insulin by 31 percent.

IF will also likely lower your risk of heart disease. It works by improving certain risk factors which include your blood sugar levels, total LDL cholesterol, blood pressure, inflammatory markers, and blood triglycerides.

As a result, it may also help prevent the occurrence of Alzheimer's disease. This neurodegenerative disease has no available cure, which makes prevention the key to delay its onset or reduce its severity. But it is likely a result of "atherosclerosis of the brain" meaning a clogging of blood vessels to the brain, very similar to that of the heart.

That being said, IF is also great for overall brain function. It boosts metabolic functions which affect the health of the brain in a positive manner. Animal studies have shown that it causes an increase in the growth of new nerve cells, attributing to greater overall brain capacity. These studies also found that this type of eating method protects the subject against brain damage after suffering from a stroke.

Fast Facts about Intermittent Fasting

To help you better understand some of the basic rudiments of the IF process, here are the most common frequently asked questions I get regarding this way of eating, and the answers I provide:

Is IF suitable for everyone?

The simple answer to this is, no. Whilst I believe (and the science shows) that intermittent fasting is perfectly safe and healthy for the vast majority of adults, there are some exceptions. You may want to avoid, or at least consult your doctor before starting an IF way of eating if you fall into one of the following groups:

- Pregnant or breastfeeding women

- You are under 18 years of age

- You have a history of serious mental health problems

- You are diabetic or taking medications for the disease

- You have recently undergone surgery

- You are suffering from a serious weight disorder

- You are underweight or malnourished

Should you exercise when you are fasting?

Yes, as we will see later on, it is actually important that you exercise during an IF program. Exercise compliments this style of eating very well, especially during the fasted state in the morning hours if weight loss in the goal.

Heavier resistance and weight training routines should ideally be performed later on in the day when adequate energy is available from the afternoon and evening meals. Again we will touch on the science and practical implications of this shortly.

Can you still undergo IF if you do not have an existing weight problem?

As stated above, IF offers many other benefits aside from just weight loss. This way of eating has a whole host of health/lifestyle benefits and is actually a very good way to develop self-control, helping a person maintain their current weight.

Does IF have any side effects?

The most obvious side effect of timing eating in this way is hunger, especially in the beginning when your body is still trying to adjust to the changes in your eating pattern. If you develop constant headaches and constipation, increase your water intake during the day. This should reduce your risk of experiencing any adverse side effects aside from hunger.

Does IF affect gout?

IF reduces inflammation, but again, make sure that you drink lots of fluid during the fasting hours. The condition can certainly worsen when a person becomes dehydrated. To reduce your risk of having gout or making it worse, avoid eating or consume a minimal amount of the following food items rich in purine: lentils, oatmeal, cauliflower, sardines, and liver.

How hungry can you get?

You will experience bouts of hunger to begin with, that's unavoidable. However you can counter this by walking, making yourself busy or drinking a calorie-free liquid. Coffee works best for me. When your body is receiving a reduced amount of calories compared to what its used to, it naturally boosts your metabolic rate. As time goes by, your body will get used to the hunger and you will know what to do to help yourself without breaking the fast. It does get easier I promise.

Why is it not advisable to those who have recently undergone an operation?

The important thing here it to give your body enough time and nutrition to heal. About 2 months for a major operation and a few weeks for a minor operation, before following any IF method. During the healing process, your body needs a constant supply of foods which are rich in micro nutrients and proteins to repair and rebuild. Whilst I have never seen adverse affects from anybody doing IF after such surgeries, it's always best to air on the side of caution until you are fully fit.

How do you maintain the weight you've lost through IF?

Once you have reached your target weight, it is recommended that you reduce the amount of days you fast per week. You can tweak the diet to suit your lifestyle. By the time you have gotten to this point, you will already be familiar with the right foods you should be eating and the proper techniques to control your cravings, to prevent yourself from overeating. Like everything else in life, discovering the best foods and times to eat them is a learning curve. Hopefully this book will give you a much better idea of how to get there.

How can you be certain that you are indeed losing weight?

It is your responsibility to monitor the changes in your weight. This is the only way you can be certain that your chosen IF method is working. However I would be careful of just monitoring the scales as the absolute measure of IF success. If you are exercising regularly you will more than likely be putting on lean muscle tissue in the process. This tissue weighs up to 3 times as much as fat, so you may not see the scales go down as fast or as much as you'd anticipated. But that's absolutely fine, as you are undergoing body recompositioning here, not just losing weight per se.

Measure your waistline as well as monitoring your weight on a weekly basis. You should find that the inches will start to fall off of the waist and hips most readily. However you may also want to measure your body fat percentage, because as I mentioned, metrics such as pure weight loss and BMI (body mass index) can be deceiving if you are gaining some lean muscle tissue in the process.

This can be measured at any doctors or health professionals office. Just about every main stream gym will now have a bioimpedance machine to calculate body fat percentage as well. Just ask one of the personal trainers if they have one to hand. I use them every week with my clients.

It is also a good idea to get them to check your resting pulse rate, blood pressure, levels of cholesterol, and fasting glucose if they can. There are devices which you can buy to perform these tests at home if required, or you can also have the tests done in a licensed clinic. This way you have a baseline reading for these metrics before you start an IF protocol. This will serve as a reference point in case you feel that something isn't going well when you do eventually start implementing a changed eating pattern.

CHAPTER 2: FASTING FOR WEIGHT LOSS & MUSCLE GAIN

"Fasting is a valid experience. It can benefit any otherwise healthy person whose calories now have the upper hand in his or her life"

(The New England Journal of Medicine)

Intermittent fasting offers many health benefits, many of which we have just discussed. However one of the main reasons many people follow the IF eating program is for the aesthetic implications. They want to do one of two things typically I.e. to lose weight or gain muscle (or both). IF proves that the usual three meals a day, breakfast, lunch, and dinner, is not a biological requirement for this, but more of a cultural artifact.

Its no secret that many people have developed an unhealthy habit of eating too much throughout the day. This gives the body an excessive supply of glucose which causes weight gain, insulin resistance, and various other health problems.

Glucose and simple sugar's are certainly not the enemy, as many people might think. They are the fuel our bodies and brains require for every task we undertake. They are essential for simply existing as a human being. However its the excess amounts of glucose which can get a person into trouble.

Fat Burning

Ultimately fasting requires you to eat less, and as a result, it reduces your caloric intake. Along with this, IF also modifies your hormonal levels. It induces the release of norepinephrine, a hormone which is accountable for burning fats in the body. Even short-term fasts can boost your metabolic rate up to 14 percent.

Following on from the fasting hours, you have to keep the first two meals of the day to a modest size. Eating a large meal to break the fast will cause your system to go into the para sympathetic mode. This will prevent the fat burning mechanisms from kicking in and will just ensure you feel tired. I will go into the specifics of exactly what to eat in terms of proposed meal plans later.

Improved Insulin/Leptin Sensitivity

A major factor of why people find it difficult to lose weight and develop obesity, is leptin resistance. Leptin sensitivity is your body's gauge on how well it is in "hearing" the signals sent by the leptin to your brain. An imbalance occurs when you supply your system with too much unhealthy food sources. The body becomes confused and tries to compensate for this, however it is possible to bring your leptin levels and sensitivity back into a normal range through improved lifestyle changes.

Leptin is known as the "fullness" hormone. Its major function is to send a signal to the brain when you have to stop eating. When you develop leptin resistance, your brain will no longer detect this signal, and you will continue eating because you believe that you are still hungry.

Eating too much processed foods and sugar causes fatty buildup in your body. These increased number of fat cells subsequently disrupt your hormone levels and lead to the production of excessive leptin. It's a vicious self-perpetuating cycle.

Lifestyle changes mean that you have to modify the way you eat and commit to a regular exercise routine in order to achieve a metabolic override. Intermittent fasting is a good choice in helping a person do this, and hence to lose weight in the process. It also shifts your system to use fat instead of sugar as the main energy source. If you are doing IF to resolve your issues with leptin resistance, eliminate fructose from your diet to help with this.

Most of your daily calories must come from healthy fats, such as nuts, olive oil, coconut oil, and avocado. Do some form of fasted cardio exercise in the morning and drink plenty of water. Make these lifestyle changes part of your daily routine and you will find it much easier to start losing those extra pounds.

Growth Hormone Response

Growth hormone (GH) is produced naturally within every normal and healthy human being. It helps your body burn fat more readily, increases the size of skeletal muscle, and makes bones stronger. GH is also capable of boosting your metabolism, slowing down the aging process and stimulating your immune system.

GH pertains to the peptide hormone, somatotropin, which is controlled by 2 hormones from the hypothalamus. These are the growth-hormone-inhibiting hormone or somatostatin and the growth-hormone-releasing hormone or somatocrinin.

A healthy lifestyle also helps in boosting the levels of your GH. It includes a healthy diet, sufficient sleep, and exercise. The most potent among these three steps is diet, but not just any kind of diet. Intermittent fasting drastically changes your eating pattern, and as a result, produces highly elevated levels of secreted GH, even while you sleep.

CHAPTER 3: FASTING FOR HEATH & LONGEVITY

"The best of all medicines are resting and fasting"

(Benjamin Franklin)

As I have already touched upon, Intermittent Fasting can be highly beneficial to a persons overall health and well-being. It does more than help you lose weight. There is a continually growing amount of evidence which is linking caloric restriction and fasting, to a reduced risk of cancers and chronic health disorders. This is greatly due to the reduction of oxidative stress on the system.

Oxidative stress coming as a result of an imbalance of antioxidative defenses (Vitamins & antioxidants) in your system, and the production of reactive free radicals. If this situation is not fixed or reduced, it may lead to a variety of health problems including liver, neurological, pulmonary, and renal diseases, as well as different kinds of cancer.

Oxidative stress is often triggered by increased body weight. Fasting prompts metabolic changes which in tern help your system adapt to the altered eating pattern. It boosts the fat oxidation to help your body maintain its composition in the given physiological range during the process. It's a double benefit, reduce weight and you reduce oxidative stress, which further improves overall health.

Better Brain Function

Recent studies by some of the world's leading scientists have concluded that fasting can greatly reduce the negative effects of aging on the brain. The process maximizes the functions of the brain because of its effective anti-inflammatory effect. These findings were proven by the researchers at the National Institute of Aging in Baltimore.

When you undergo the process of IF, your body will experience two phases which will result in greater overall brain function. These major phases are building and cleansing. The building phase occurs when you eat. The hormone insulin stimulates the body to update nutrition into the body via the food we eat. This is what is described as an anabolic process. However this process isn't very selective in the sense that the body will begin to store not only nutrients, but toxins also. The body will utilize these stored elements to build new tissues and cells. It will also keep nutrients where the body will get its energy from at times when you don't eat I.e. muscle and liver glycogen stores.

The cleansing phase occurs when you fast for more than six hours. This phase is catabolic in nature I.e. a breaking down process. The old and damaged cells are torn apart. It prompts the brain to turn on its autophagy or "self-eating" mode. As a result, the body releases human growth hormone which activates the genetic repair mechanisms. The cells work by regulating these waste materials, before beginning this repair process on themselves.

This is an innate mechanism which aids in boosting your body's natural immunity. It also enhances tissue healing and reduces inflammation, again quite critically with regards to the brain.

Intermittent fasting has also shown to improve the levels of a person's Brain-Derived NeuroTrophic Factor (BDNF). This substance leads to the development of new synapses and neuron pathways within the brain. This also results in improved communication between the cells of the brain and existing healthy neurons, in a process known as "neuroplasticity".

However when the levels of BDNF are low, the reverse occurs. The brain encounters processing problems linked to various problems which include memory loss, dementia, and eventually Alzheimer's.

Cancer Prevention and Treatment

Cancer is unfortunately still among the leading causes of mortality in the world. Over the past 30 years or so, the available treatment for the disease remains relatively unchanged. There are still no clear guidelines with regards to the nutrition which may affect the incidence of cancer, although there is no doubt that what we eat has a large part to play in the likelihood of developing the disease.

Meanwhile, the dietary recommendation for patients who are undergoing chemotherapy, according to the American Cancer Society, is the increased intake of protein and calories to help maintain size and strength.

There are ongoing preliminary and preclinical studies on the role of fasting and dietary restriction in prompting chemotherapy resistance and cellular protection. Both fasting and calorie restriction have shown beneficial effects in the effectiveness of cancer therapies and in the prevention of malignancies.

The interest in intermittent fasting for cancer prevention and treatment started way back in 1945. It was during this time when one of the first major studies on the topic was conducted. It illustrated that the process of fasting aids in reducing the occurrence of breast cancer tumors in rats and extended their lifespan as a result. A more recent study in 2009 proved that IF can reduce the negative side effects of the chemotherapy process.

Valter Longo, an associate professor of biology and gerontology at USC who contributed to the recent study, suggested the results of the process was mainly due to how the body and cells react when fasting, and that the system goes into a starvation mode. He suggests that although the cancerous tumors do not stop growing when the body starves, fasting in general affects the healthy cells by boosting their stress resistance. As a result, these healthy cells are able to withstand the chemotherapy process compared with the unhealthy cells.

Longo continued with these studies and after a few years, he concluded that many types of cancer in mice can be cured by fasting alone. During the process, the healthy cells go into a hibernation mode while the cancer cells try to spread but fail. These unhealthy cells try to find what's missing in the blood after fasting. They try to replace the missing elements but fail.

This doesn't mean that IF will work in preventing and curing cancer the same in humans, but does suggest a beneficial path to perhaps take. Fasting is not recommended to cancer patients who have developed chronic diseases and have already dropped 10 percent (or more) of their body weight.

Always make sure that you consult a physician before starting out with any diet plan. Different patients have varying nutrition requirements depending on the gravity of their condition and how well their bodies are responding to the illness and treatment.

The effects of intermittent fasting on cancer prevention have yet to gather sufficient scientific findings. There is big potential in this area, and the initial studies indicate a lot of promise due to the positive results of the experiments done thus far.

However always remember that the effects of fasting vary depending on many factors, such as your baseline health and energy levels. It is not easy. It is mind over matter most of the time. It is also not recommended for everyone, especially those who are pregnant or breastfeeding, and those who are diabetic and hypoglycemic.

But to the average everyday person, intermittent fasting promotes health and longevity in a number of ways. It gives you a chance to get back in shape, maintain your weight, and live a healthier life. It's all about self-discipline. It's about following a healthy lifestyle and being selective with what you eat, and just as importantly, when to eat it.

PART 2: INTERMITTENT FASTING - PRACTICAL TIPS FOR IMPLEMENTING ON A DAILY BASIS

CHAPTER 4: THE DIFFERENT INTERMITTENT FASTING DAILY SCHEDULES/METHODS

"One of the reasons intermittent fasting can work is that is reconnects you with what hunger feels like"

(Chris Mohn)

So having discussed the main health and fitness considerations when it comes to fasting. It's now time to take a look at the various methods a person can put intermittent fasting into action on a daily basis. Everyone will have a slightly different preference on how to do this simply due to their current lifestyle, but most can be worked into the average persons schedule without too much hassle.

There are six popular methods of intermittent fasting in general. These methods vary with regards to schedules/timing depending on the targets and goals of the individual. The effectiveness of each method again depends on the person, and their discipline in sticking with the protocol. So make sure that you choose the type which fits you best, in terms of goals, health, and lifestyle.

16/8 Method (Leangains)

The 16/8 fasting protocol is probably the most well know and widely used IF method today. It was popularized by fitness expert Martin Berkhan, and restricts your eating window to 8 to 10 hours per day. This is actually perceived by many as the most natural fasting method. It requires 14 to 15 hours of daily fasting for women and 16 hours for men. To make matters easier if you are following this method, simply skip breakfast and do not eat anything after dinner. You can eat 2 to 3 large meals within the eating window.

This method is easier for people who usually skip breakfast, but a tough challenge for those who get hungry at the start of their day. If you are among the latter, I assure you that a few days acclimatization is all it takes to get used to, just make sure you have some coffee on hand, especially in the beginning.

Sample schedule:

- If you had your last meal at 8 in the evening, you have to restrict yourself from eating until 12 noon the following day.

- You simply have to count up to 16 hours of fasting before eating your next meal.

- During the fast, you can reduce your hunger levels by drinking non-caloric beverages, coffee, and water.

- During your eating window, nourish yourself by eating healthy, satiating foods. Avoid too much highly processed junk foods.

Eat-Stop-Eat

This is one of the most popular fasting methods popularized by fitness expert Brad Pilon. It requires a 24-hour fast at least once or twice per week. This schedule can be fairly difficult for the beginner to IF. Help yourself by starting with the Leangains method if this is your first try at fasting. Allow your system time to get used to the habit of not eating for a period of time before trying this method.

Sample schedule:

- To achieve a 24-hour fast, you simply have to stop eating from the time of your last meal up to the same time the following day.

- For example, if you finished your last meal on Sunday at 8pm in the evening, refrain from eating until 8pm the following day.

- Choose fasting days which fit your schedule. You can do them at times when you are not particularly busy or when you are traveling for instance.

- It is not necessary to fast from dinner to dinner. You can do it from breakfast to breakfast or from lunch to lunch.

- During the fasting hours, you cannot eat anything solid but can drink water, non-caloric drinks, and coffee.

- Eat in a regular fashion during your eating periods I.e. do not drastically over eat.

This method requires more self-discipline than the 16/8 method. Expect the last hours of the fast to be extra difficult as you will become extremely hungry, although it will get easier to deal with over time.

5:2 Diet (Fast Diet)

This method of fasting popularized by doctor and British journalist Michael Mosley, allows you to eat a full amount of calories for 5 days and then restrict your caloric intake to 500 to 600 for 2 days. You are free to choose the two days when you will restrict the amount of calories that you take based on preference and schedule.

Sample schedule:

- Eat in a regular fashion during the week, then on the weekends (Saturdays and Sundays) reduce your eating to just two small meals a day.

- You can also choose two days which are not consecutive to make it easier to perform. As you get used to the process, you can change this schedule back to a fasting period of two consecutive days if you wish.

- It is easier to hit about 500 calories at a time during your fasting day than to divide the amount by eating small snacks throughout the day. Choosing the latter will make you feel unsatisfied and will increase the chances of failing with the method.

The Warrior Diet

This fasting method popularized by fitness expert Ori Hofmekler, requires fasting during the day and eating all you want at night. It is somewhat similar to the carbohydrate back-loading method I will detail in a later chapter, but a little more extreme.

Sample schedule:

- The fasting period happens for up to 20 hours, leaving you with 3 to 5 hours of eating window at dinner time.

- This IF style offers the most benefits among all the fasting methods, but is also one of the most extreme.

- While you are still trying to adjust, you can snack on some fruits or veggies during the day. After a while, stick to the rule and consume only water, coffee, or tea within your fasting hours.

- The most important thing in this scheme is to stay hydrated during the day.

- Eat nutrient and caloric dense foods during the feast part of the diet. Focus on whole foods with a balanced amount of fats, protein, and carbohydrates.

- To hit your total goals, it will help to snack on nuts, cottage cheese, seeds, or a protein shake before bed.

The food choices in this method are similar to the food list of the Paleo diet. You have to choose foods which are whole and unprocessed.

Alternate-Day Fasting

As the name suggests, this method of IF requires you to fast every other day. This means going all-out hungry as you go to bed several times a week. This method is not recommended for beginners. It is very similar to the Eat-Stop-Eat protocol, however the person will be fasting for 3-4 days in a week, as opposed to just 2 24 hour periods.

Sample schedule:

- You can choose to begin any day you want and fast the next day.

- During your fasting days, you can choose not to eat or consume about 500 calories.

- Make sure that you stay hydrated during your fasting days

by drinking lots of water. You may also drink caffeinated beverages such as tea or coffee to keep energy levels and attentiveness high.

Spontaneous Meal Skipping

This method of fasting does not follow a rigid plan like the previous protocols I have listed. You simply have to skip meals whenever it is convenient. You can opt to skip a meal or two when you don't have time to eat or whenever you are not hungry.

This method disproves the myth that people must eat every few hours or else they will lose muscle or go into a catabolic starvation mode. The fact is, the human body is capable of handling famine for a long period of time, and as we've already seen, actually thrives when it is forced into this state.

Skipping meals won't cause any harm. As with all of these IF methods, nourish yourself with healthy foods during the hours when you are not fasting and you will not have any problems. If you do things correctly, you should simply experience the multitude of health and detox/cleansing benefits which come along with such an eating strategy.

CHAPTER 5: FOOD EXAMPLES AND MEAL PLANS

"More caution and perhaps more restraint are necessary in breaking a fast than in keeping it"

(Mahatma Gandhi)

IF is not merely a diet, but an eating schedule which brings a whole host of health benefits when practiced regularly. Everything from the acceleration of weight (fat) loss, muscle growth and a plethora of health and lifestyle benefits. IF is something you have already been doing but you are not aware of. You voluntarily fast when you sleep. When you sleep, the fasting interval constitutes the duration of time between your last meal at night, up to your first meal in the morning. This is where the term breakfast came about. It is the first meal of the day which is intended to "break the fast."

The old way of doing things was to eat in a conventional pyramid in terms of your meal sizes. It would look something like this:

Eat Supper like a beggar

Eat Dinner Like a Pauper

Eat Lunch Like a Prince

Eat Breakfast Like a King

This theory was based on outdated metabolism models which suggest that the body only has time to burn off calories when the person is awake. So better off getting most of your calories in the morning when you have the rest of the day to burn them off.

However as we will see later on with regards to insulin activity, this is almost the worst thing you can do, especially if weight loss is your goal. Essentially increased insulin sensitivity first thing in the morning ensures a person will store much more of these calories as adipose tissue (fat stores). It is also preventing the person from tapping into existing fat stores by inhibiting a fasting state. It's a double whammy.

In reality, the way in which the body works from a hormonal and metabolism standpoint, is the reverse of what your parents told you. The old portion size pyramid should actually be inverted I.e:

Eat Supper Like a King
Eat Dinner Like a Prince
Eat lunch Like a Pauper
Eat Breakfast like a beggar

This is especially relevant when it comes carbohydrates and simple sugars. I will get into this in greater depth when exploring the considerations of carbohydrate backloading, which ties in very closely with intermittent fasting. Regular 16:8 IF removes all calories in the AM, whilst backloading removes the carbohydrates and sugars, but leaves some room for proteins.

The good news is that the inverted portion pyramid actually fits into most people's lifestyle habits very easily. The majority of people will eat breakfast alone, so cutting it down considerably, or removing the meal altogether, is very doable. This affords them the opportunity to go to lunch with friends and certainly dinner. But more importantly to be able to enjoy what they are eating when they do I.e. not calorie restrict or always pick the "healthiest" option.

Saying that, it is still advisable to keep the first two meals (especially the first one around lunch time) to a modest healthy portion.

Breaking your fast with a big meal shifts your body from a super charged, sympathetic autonomic nervous system state (where you are burning calories and fat) to a lethargic parasympathetic state where your body has switched to a "rest & digest" state (forcing a big insulin response to store calories as opposed to metabolizing them). It will also make you tired throughout the afternoon.

The trick is to eat enough to give you some energy and provide the body with some fuel and nutrients it needs, but no more. Never overtax your digestive system, especially after the fasting hours. Again eat enough to satisfy your hunger but never too much. Begin with meals which contain around 400-500 calories. Here are some sample meals that you can have to break the fast:

- 1 apple, 1 can of tuna, and 1 tablespoon of olive oil

- A handful of berries and omelet (2 whole eggs, plus 2 egg whites)

- Cottage cheese or Greek yogurt, served with almonds and berries

- 1 cup of unsweetened almond milk, mixed with 40 grams of whey protein, and 20 grams of almonds, and a serving of fruit

- 1 apple, salad greens, 1/2 avocado, and chicken breast

The key to nutrition when you are on this kind of diet is to include healthy fats, fruit, and a convenient source of protein. Aside from being nutritious, fruits are easily digestible and can replenish glycogen in the liver. When your system gets an ample supply of liver glycogen, you will experience reduced hunger as your body enters the anabolic state.

After the first 2 small meals, you can eat more in order to keep up with the required caloric intake depending on your goals. Your meals must have moderate amounts of carbohydrates and fats, and a high amount of protein. If you are already having a fatty slice of meat, such as salmon or beef, refrain from adding fats to your meal. If you are having chicken, which is a leaner source of protein, you can add fats sparingly. You can opt to use coconut oil for cooking, serve the meat with steamed rice or potatoes, and top them with cheese.

Honestly, the great thing about IF is this evening meal. You have the ability to eat much more liberally in terms of both portion size and choice of food. You can afford to consume around 1000-1200 calories for this meal. The body is able to intake and metabolize food with much higher efficiency due to it being primed by the fast earlier in the day. This even allows you to get away with small amounts of "junk food" here. However if weight loss is your goal, you may still want to stick to the somewhat healthier options even at dinner time. The following is a list of some sample meals you can follow:

- 1 chicken breast, 100 grams of pasta, vegetables, favorite dressing

- A large salmon/tuna steak, brown rice, vegetables, squeezed lemon

- Beef steak, potato wedges/sweet potato, vegetables, mushroom/black pepper sauce

Practical Tips to Make IF Work

There are three important factors that you have to take into account when you follow any method of intermittent fasting:

1. What do you eat?

2. When do you eat?

3. How can you adapt fasting into your lifestyle?

Always remember an important rule of intermittent fasting: eat like an adult. This means that on the days or hours when you are not fasting, you have to eat real food. Choose smart carbohydrates you can get from fruits, vegetables, rice, oats, and many more. It is okay to indulge in your favorite treats, like cakes, cookies, and other sweets, once in a while so that you won't feel deprived.

Eat slow. Always be mindful of how fast you are eating. Chew your food and taste every mouthful. People have a tendency to scoff down food too quickly after a period of fasting as they are super hungry. But the trick is to just treat the meal as if you would during a regular 2-3 hour eating pattern.

On a similar note, enjoy your food but do not overeat. Stop after you have reached your daily nutrient requirement on fasting days, or once you are already full on regular days. Make this part of your lifestyle. Again this isn't some fad diet, intermittent fasting is something to incorporate into your day for the long term, and it is only difficult in the beginning. Make every step a daily habit and you will soon get used to it. Just like brushing your teeth, everything will feel like a routine eventually.

If a routine sounds like a bore, you can tweak and spice things up so that you will not end up eating the same thing over and over again. One of the main benefits of this style of eating (or any healthy plan) is that it allows you to eat an unlimited amount of vegetables. Here are some of the best ways to prepare your veggies:

1. Steamed – There are many vegetables which taste great when steamed, including broccoli, peppers, carrots, asparagus, onion, and cauliflower. This is certainly your healthiest and lowest fat option when it comes to preparation and cooking style.

2. Roasted – Place sliced veggies on a baking tray lined with aluminum foil. Lightly spray with olive oil and season the veggies with salt and pepper. Bake them for 30 minutes in a preheated oven at 250 degrees. Some of the best veggies that you can roast include sprouts, cauliflower, sweet potatoes, and broccoli.

3. Cauliflower rice. Chop the cauliflower and put the pieces into a blender or food processor. Process until the consistency is similar to that of rice. Heat a tablespoon of oil in a skillet over medium heat. Saute the cauliflower rice for a few minutes. Cover the skillet and leave to steam for 8 minutes. Season with salt and pepper before serving.

4. Prosciutto wrapped asparagus. Wrap two pieces of asparagus with half a slice of prosciutto. Lightly spray with olive oil and bake for 20 minutes in a preheated oven at 250 degrees.

5. Barbecue. Put your preferred vegetable slices on a skewer. You can use peppers, zucchini, baby tomatoes, onions and many more. Marinate them in olive oil and season with salt and pepper before grilling.

6. French fried. Slice your veggies into thin and long strips. You can use white potatoes, sweet potatoes, parsnips, or carrots. Put the sliced veggies in a Ziploc bag. Season with olive oil and your preferred spice. You can use cumin, cinnamon, rosemary, or chili powder. Bake in a preheated oven at 275 degrees until crispy.

Good Sources of Fats

You need to nourish yourself with a balanced supply of carbohydrates, protein, and other essential nutrients. You also have to load up with a good amount of healthy fats. I have covered some of these in the previous meal plan ideas, but here are some of the best fat sources you can include in your meals:

- Avocados

- Nuts and seeds

- Cottage Cheese

- Coconut and coconut oil

- Olives and olive oil

- Nut butters (peanut & almond)

Best Protein Sources

Make sure that you are also including protein in all of your main meals, which you can get from a broad range of sources including the following:

- Seafood. Include as much seafood as you can in your meals. Some of the best choices of seafood are tuna, mussels, salmon, shrimp, scallops, and tilapia.

- Animal protein. You can use a lot of meat including ground meat and the darker types, but more sparingly then the leaner white meats. Some good sources of protein include ham, bison, beef, turkey, and chicken.

- Dairy products. Serve the right portion of dairy in your meals. You can choose from a variety of products which include high protein/low fat sources such as Greek yogurt, goat yogurt, eggs, cottage cheese, skimmed milk, and ricotta.

The most important thing to remember is that you have to eat quality whole food. Prepare your meals in a variety of ways, spice them up, and enjoy the process.

Low-Carb Food that You Can Incorporate in Your Daily Meal Plan

To make things easier for you when planning your meals, here's a more detailed list of what you can mix and match to meet your daily nutrient requirement when undergoing intermittent fasting:

1. Seafood and fish. Most of these sources contain little or no carbs at all, and are rich in vitamin B12, omega-3 fatty acids, and iodine.

- Sardines

- Salmon

- Shellfish

- Trout

- Haddock

- Tuna

- Herring

- Catfish

- Halibut

- Cod

- Lobster

2. Eggs. Eggs are some of the most nutritious foods that you can prepare in a variety of ways. They contain zero carbohydrate content and are loaded with nutrients and micro nutrients which are beneficial to the brain and eyes.

3. Vegetables. Avoid eating starchy root vegetables, such as potatoes and sweet potatoes, because they contain high amounts of carbs. You can choose from the following healthy veggies that are suited for this kind of diet:

- Broccoli

- Tomatoes

- Onions

- Cauliflower

- Brussels Sprouts

- Cucumber

- Kale

- Asparagus

- Eggplant

- Green beans

- Bell Peppers

- Mushrooms

- Zucchini

- Cabbage

- Swiss chard

- Celery

- Spinach

4. Meats. Almost every kind of animal product will contain little or no carbs. You can eat bacon but only in moderation. Avoid the brands of bacon that are cured in sugar and contain a lot of preservatives. Instead you should opt for:

- Beef

- Lamb

- Chicken

- Bison

- Veal

- Turkey

- Venison

5. Fats and oils. Avoid unhealthy and refined vegetable oils, such as soybean oil and corn oil. Choose any of the following healthy oils:

- Extra virgin olive oil

- Coconut oil

- Avocado oil

6. Fruits and berries. Most fruit sources contain more simple sugars than vegetables. Eat only a couple of servings each day for the micro nutrients they provide. This is especially true of high fructose containing fruits as the body is unable to utilize these as energy, and only metabolized by the liver. The following sources however are OK to indulge on:

- Strawberries

- Avocado

- Olives

- Apricots

7. Nuts and seeds. Essentially humans should be eating much more of these food sources than we currently do. Nuts and seeds are a great source vitamins, minerals, fiber, fats & protein.

- Coconuts

- Almonds

- Macadamia nuts

- Peanuts

- Chia seeds

- Walnuts

- Hazelnuts

- Sunflower seeds

- Flax seeds

- Cashews

- Pistachios

- Pumpkin seeds

8. Condiments and herbs. The one thing you want to avoid during a healthy eating plan is continually consuming foods which are too bland. This can throw a person of the schedule quicker than anything I've noticed. The key is to use healthy condiments in

moderation, some of which include the following:

- Pepper

- Cinnamon

- Salt

- Garlic

- Oregano

- Mustard

9. Dark chocolate. If there is one guilty pleasure I allow myself to indulge in its this. Dark chocolate is actually considered a health food and is known to reduce your risk of heart problems and lower your blood pressure. It also aids in boosting brain function due to its high antioxidant content. Go for the brands with 80 percent or more cocoa if you can.

10. Beverages. Avoid fruit juices which are loaded with sugars and glucose. Choose from the following drinks to keep yourself hydrated and keep your mind off the hunger:

- Water

- Carbonated water/Club soda (with no added sugar)

- Coffee

- Tea

Other Tips to Help Your Fasting Success

Remember the following tips which should make your life easier when attempting to start on any of the methods of IF we have covered here. The most important thing is to just stick with it:

1. Check your schedule and plans before starting the eating plan. It is better to schedule most of the fasting hours at night while you sleep. This will elevate your chances of success as you reduce the time you will be thinking about food, reducing your cravings, and avoiding temptations.

2. Drink plenty of water, especially during the fasting hours, to keep yourself hydrated. Drink water on an empty stomach upon waking each morning. The reason why you are hungry first thing is the lack of water intake while you were sleeping. If your goal is to lose weight, drink at least half a liter of water in the morning. Throughout the day, drink at least another 2 liters of water for women and up to 4 liters for men.

3. Taking BCAAs while you are on this kind of eating plan can speed up the weight loss process. BCAAs are the branched-chain amino acids or the three important amino acids which have a special branched structure. These amino acids are leucine, valine, and isoleucine.

Ingesting BCAAs while you are on a low-calorie diet will make it easier for your system to lose visceral fat. This is especially helpful to people who are consistently training as BCAA consumption also reduces muscle breakdown. By taking about 12 grams of BCAAs each day while you are on an IF style plan, you will be supplying your body with the base essential building blocks it requires to recover, build lean muscle tissue as well as supporting hormonal and immune function.

4. Exercise. I will cover this in greater depth in a following chapter. However physical activity, both the type and timing, are key to complimenting an IF type eating plan to reach ones goals. Hint: This will usually consist of moderate cardiovascular exercise in the AM whilst in a fasted state, and heavier resistance type workouts later in the afternoon/evening when there is greater nutritional fuel in the system.

5. Have an ample supply of stock cubes. This may seem like an odd suggestion, but they will come in handy at times when you can no longer control your hunger. You can take the cube and mix with water to make a basic soup. The idea is to have a very simple and low calorie drink with some flavor to stave off any major hunger pangs. You may even just want to cut the cube in half. It is ideal to take this before going to bed so that your mind will stop thinking about food and hunger.

6. Aside from water, you can drink tea or coffee anytime during the day. Caffeine is a natural appetite suppressant. Take these drinks in moderation as having too much caffeine can make you feel

anxious. Also, avoid drinking them a couple of hours before you sleep at night to avoid disrupting sleep as best you can.

CHAPTER 6: INTERMITTENT FASTING EXERCISE PROTOCOLS

This book was not intended to be a workout guide by any measure, it's about educating you on the considerations of intermittent fasting, and how best to put these principles into place. However it would be remiss of me not to outline some of the most beneficial workout routines which compliment IF so well. To discuss some of the exercise principles (type & timing) which help people reach their goals with this way of eating.

So the following is a brief overview of what I myself do, and advise my clients to do also. Much like the food plans, what I like about intermittent fasting exercise plans is that they remain relatively similar regardless of your objectives. They just vary with regards to intensity and duration. Let me explain what I mean.

Essentially what you are looking to do is maximize your fat loss potential in the morning in your fasted state. This means performing some form of cardiovascular activity after you have woken up, and before you eat your first meal.

This might be light walking if you are simply trying to lose a little weight. It might be heavy jogging/cycling if you are trying to lose a lot. Again it just comes down to your current body weight/composition and fitness goals.

If your intention is to put on some lean muscle mass, you will have to incorporate a training session to stimulate this growth. A resistance/weight training workout which is more optimally saved until the afternoon or evening time, when you have some more energy and fuel to sustain such activities. Some people can workout with moderate to heavy weights in the morning, but most people (myself included) struggle with this.

If your goal is to gain muscle mass, which it should be for both male and females, then you should always include a weight training routine at least 3 times a week. For guys its usually a given, but for girls, they have a tendency to skip these workouts. They buy into the myth that resistance work will make them "bulky".

Again, I do not want to turn this book into a discussion on exercise science & muscle hypertrophy etc but nothing could be further from the truth. Females do not become big by lifting weights. They lean out and gain a better overall body composition and posture.

I know what a lot of people will now be thinking. "I don't have time to workout twice a day!" I understand this would be the case for most people within our hectic lives. However this is why intermittent fasting is so beneficial and effective, as it cuts down the amount of physical work a person needs to perform.

A brief walk in the morning most days and evening workouts in the gym 3 times a week will usually do it. I have included some very general physical activity protocols to follow below. These are designed to give you a baseline knowledge, some guidance on how best to structure your day for optimal results when intermittent fasting. You can then incorporate your own workouts either yourself or with your personal trainer.

Beginner/Low Fitness Level/Weight loss Goals

AM - 20 mins light walk/cycle/swim (Every other day)

PM - 30 min resistance workout (3 times a week)

Intermediate/Moderate Fitness Level/Weight loss Goals + Muscle Growth

AM - 30 minute moderate walk/cycle/swim (5 times a week)

PM - 45 min resistance workout (4 times a week)

Advanced/High Fitness Level/Weight loss Goals + Muscle Growth

AM - 45 minute moderate walk/cycle/swim (Every day)

PM - 1 hour resistance workout (5 times a week)

Note that the intensity of morning cardiovascular activity never gets above a moderate level in terms of intensity. This is due to the considerations of oxidization of certain energy substrates. Remember the goal here is fat burning. This is achieved at low to moderate intensities when the oxidative ratios or P/O (Phosphate/Oxygen) ratio is optimal for burning fat molecules.

To ensure this, heart rate must stay in a medium range. If intensity and heart rate raise too high and too quickly, you cannot get enough oxygen into the system to support the metabolism of fatty molecules. The body will simply switch to burning the most easily oxidized and readily available energy source I.e. carbohydrates in the form blood sugar and muscle glycogen, as this can be done with lower levels of oxygen within the blood stream.

If you are attempting to increase your overall fitness levels, then I would leave the high intensity sprint work until later in the day. Again the goal early in the day is fat loss, not an increase in cardiovascular capacity or athletic performance per se.

Of course if you have any health concerns regarding physical activity and exercise, you should always consult your doctor before taking on such a program. The above is just an outline with regards to the science and real world observations I've made over the years, for getting optimal results whilst eating on an IF type schedule.

CHAPTER 7: CARBOHYDRATE BACKLOADING

While the considerations of carbohydrate manipulation is a discussion in and of itself, in my opinion its one which ties in very closely with intermittent fasting. This is why I have included a chapter on carbohydrate backloading within this book.

Both strategies are essentially making best use of the bodies natural hormonal cycles and rhythms to aid a person in achieving their health and fitness goals, which is usually to get/stay lean whilst holding onto or building as much lean muscle tissue as possible.

I mentioned within the introduction that it was possible to have your cake and eat it with regards to weight loss, health and eating, if you know what you are doing. If you know how to time things correctly. I use a combination of IF and carbohydrate backloading to maintain an 8-10% body fat year round whilst almost eating what I want.

The key is carbohydrates and the timing of their consumption. Most people believe carbs to be the enemy, however nothing could be further from the truth. Carbohydrates are broken down into glucose and then glycogen, the number one substrate our bodies use to fuel everything, from movement to thinking.

The problem is when people consume too much, they begin to convert and store this excess glycogen as fat. However they need this carbohydrate energy source to get big and strong. On the flip side, a big reduction in carb intake will see the person lose weight, but find it very difficult to maintain and build muscle in the process (as well as always having a general lack of energy).

So how do you eat enough carbs for energy and muscle growth without putting on excess fat? Like IF, its about timing. More specifically its about insulin sensitivity timing. When you consume a carbohydrate heavy meal, the excess blood sugars trigger an insulin response and a signal for the body to uptake and store those carbs where it can. This will either be as liver/muscle glycogen or adipose tissue (fat stores) if the former are full.

So when is insulin sensitivity at its highest? There are two time periods predominantly. The first is in the morning when you first wake up. This is why I suggested that the inverted food portion pyramid works so well. Any food, and especially sugary or starchy carbs ingested at breakfast, will largely by absorbed and stored where ever the body can.

The second time when insulin sensitivity is high is immediately after heavy physical activity I.e. a resistance workout with weights for example. So taking this into consideration, how should you be timing your carbohydrate consumption?

As the name suggests, you need to be "backloading" these carbs in the latter part of the day. Avoid them in the morning when insulin sensitivity is high, if you are intermittent fasting this is not a problem as you are only drinking water or coffee. If you are carbohydrate backloading then you should only be consuming a high protein meal such as an egg omelette or protein shake etc.

The same should be followed at lunch time I.e. a high protein/ moderate fat meal consisting of foods already mentioned in the meal plans in an earlier chapter. This will again ensure no excess uptake of carbohydrates into the system.

Now here is the key. To make the best use of carbohydrate backloading, you need to make use of an afternoon workout. The most optimal time of day to do this is around 3-5pm when insulin sensitivity starts to wear off. However a heavy resistance type workout will actually kick it back into gear.

Now you have just had the benefit of working out fasted (which will burn excess fat) and it will also further deplete muscle glycogen stores which is the key to this working. After the workout you are free to eat anything you would like, including almost all of the sugary and starchy carbs you would like, up until bed time.

The reason you will not store any of these carbs as fat, even though you have just created a new insulin spike, is due to muscle glycogen stores being low or empty. So what the body does is shuttle these energy substrates straight back into the muscles to replenish the glycogen stores, ready for the next days workout. People will often find they can eat ice-cream, doughnuts, literally anything with this method and wake up the next morning even leaner than the night before!

Now I know that it might not be feasible for everyone to workout in the afternoon, but it is possible to manipulate this a little by going to the gym in the early evening around 6-8pm. The concept still works.

The basic premise is to either consume no, or very few carbs in the morning/early afternoon before your workout, and load back up on them in the evening after your workout. Again much like IF, carbohydrate backloading works so well in that it not only runs alongside the bodies natural hormonal cycles, it also works with their lifestyle and social life patterns as well. It allows people to eat as much of and what ever they like whilst out for dinner with friends etc.

There is only one drawback to this way of scheduling carbs, which I have already touched upon within in earlier chaper, and that is having enough fuel in the system and energy to get a good resistance style workout in. I must admit, I sometimes struggle without any carbs before I train, so always add in around 30-50 grams for lunch on heavy training days.

However some people are OK to train just fine on zero carbs before working out. The carbs they eat the night before sufficiently loaded their muscle glycogen stores, which is the predominant fuel source you will be using during the workout anyway. On non training days, just follow a similar eating schedule I.e. little/no carbs until your evening meals.

They trick to all of this is to test these strategies out for yourself and see what your body responds to best. Then you can adapt things from there depending on how you feel and the results you are achieving. Whether that is utilizing a full IF program to eradicate all calories in the morning, or you are simply consuming proteins. The approaches are very similar in nature.

The premise is the same, stay away from sugary carbohydrates when either insulin sensitivity is high or muscle/liver glycogen stores are full. This will ensure that the body does not store these carbs as fat deposits on the body, but instead uses them to replenish energy stores in order to fuel your workouts.

SUMMARY

The first thing I always look for when studying some exercise or nutrition concept, is the body of evidence which supports it. To look for the science behind why it should work, and to make sense of it from a physiological standpoint. Then I see if this translates into practice in the real world. To see if I myself, and my clients are attaining the positive results the theory suggests we should be getting.

Intermittent fasting is no different. On paper it comes with so many health and fitness benefits, that it would be remiss of us not to test. In fact, it is not really a new concept at all, everyone from our earliest ancestors practiced fasting (out of necessity) to more recent thinkers over the past 2000 years (out of choice).

These individuals could certainly see the benefits such an eating style brings, in terms of the way they looked and felt. Today it is simply about choosing a style and method of IF which best fits into your schedule. For most people this will be the 18:6 method, where an over night fast is extended throughout the morning hours.

The most difficult adjustment for most people is skipping breakfast. We were all told that a big healthy breakfast is the way to go. So the first few days transitioning to intermittent fasting will be tough without these calories in the AM. But once your body has adjusted, it will start to get used to it and thrive in this fasted state.

Coffee is the key for me. Coffee will not only get you though the initial hunger pangs you will almost certainly experience, but it will also speed up your metabolism, helping you burn off excess fat even quicker. I have 2 cups throughout the morning to keep me going. You may prefer tea or some other source of caffeine for this.

Then you are free to eat liberally throughout the afternoon and into the evening time. Try to keep this first meal light when breaking your fast. You do not want to shift your body straight back into an anabolic state right away. Ease yourself in with a healthy 400-500 calorie meal to kick your metabolism back into gear.

Then slowly increase meal size throughout the day, which usually means culminating in a large feast for dinner to satisfy your satiation for the foods you enjoy. Only this time without the guilt, as you have earned those calories through you fast earlier in the day.

In reality it all comes down to hormonal activity, and more specifically insulin sensitivity. If you know how the body works from this standpoint, it will not be difficult to make the adjustment in eating, as it will seem logical now. Invert that outdated meal portion pyramid and you will be just fine.

Then it is about complementing this eating style with the right physical activity and exercise protocol. It's about exploiting this early morning fasted state with low to moderate cardiovascular exercise to further deplete liver and muscle glycogen stores, forcing your body into burning its excess fat stores for fuel. Save the intense resistance and muscle building routines until the afternoon, when you have more energy to get them done.

This is the protocol I myself follow, as well as the clients I coach on a daily basis. Whether they are following an 18:6 IF plan or carbohydrate backloading, the concept remains the same. Eat little to nothing in the morning, and go big in the evening. It's simply about trying these routines out for yourself to see what works best in terms of your own body, goals and lifestyle.

CONCLUSION

"Fasts don't have to be scary. They are just another tool on your tool belt"

(Dave Smith)

So there you have it. A complete guide on how intermittent fasting works, and more importantly, how it can work for you. If this is your first time coming across this method of meal scheduling, it might seem strange, even counterintuitive. But I assure you that the science works in your favor if you do decide to give it a go.

To others this will come more naturally, especially if you are used to skipping meals, particularly breakfast. For some, just a coffee in the morning will naturally do for them. For these people its simply about incorporating the right exercise programs into their day to optimize this morning fasted state.

So just go ahead and see what works best for you. But make sure you give it a real go. As I always tell my clients, I can give you the information, but nothing will work unless you do! So whatever you decide to do, I wish you every success with your health and fitness goals in this life.

All the best.